Fibromyalgia

A NUTRITIONAL APPROACH

William Hennen, Ph.D.

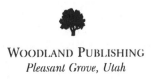

WOODLAND PUBLISHING
Pleasant Grove, Utah

© 1999
Woodland Publishing, Inc.
P.O. Box 160
Pleasant Grove, Utah
84062

Contents

Introduction

Fibromyalgia (FM) is a syndrome characterized by widespread musculoskeletal pain and tenderness at specified sites, fatigue, and unrefreshing sleep.[1] Fibromyalgia (FM) afflicts predominantly middle-aged women.[2] Research investigations have shown a disturbed microcirculation in painful muscles, a decrease in adenosine triphosphate and phosphocreatine, and a reduced relaxation rate. Pain analyses indicate that the pain is nociceptive, meaning that there is an abnormally high pain sensitivity. A characteristic physiological sleep disturbance is also one of the main symptoms of FM. The cause(s) of FM is not known, though it may be different in different patients. FM is a clinical entity, but should be regarded as a syndrome rather than a disease.[3]

Fibromyalgia is classified as a syndrome rather than a disease.[4] The difference between a syndrome and a disease is that a disease is a condition with a clearly identifiable causative agent while a syndrome is a set of symptoms which define the condition without a single consistent causative agent upon which to place the blame. Thus a cold is a disease because a viral infection can be identified as the causative agent.

Fibromyalgia is a syndrome because the identifiable factors vary even though the symptoms are present. This can be likened to the operation of a car. A car will not run if its gas tank is empty. On the other hand a car with a full gas tank still will not run if its battery is dead. Thus a whole list of functions must be present for a car to run properly while the absence of any one function is sufficient to prevent the car from running. The human body is infinitely more complex than a car and many more functions must be working properly for the body to operate efficiently. The body unlike the car has an interest in its own well-being. The body has many self-healing mechanisms and many self-compensating mechanisms. If given the right the tools, sufficient time, and correct instructions the body can heal itself.

Comorbidities

Fibromyalgia has also been found to be related to a number of other conditions including chronic fatigue immune deficiency syndrome (CFIDS),[5] major depressive disorder[6], myofascial pain syndrome,[7] Sjogren's syndrome,[8] irritable bowel syndrome,[9] temporamandibular joint (TMJ) syndrome,[10] premenstrual syndrome (PMS), tensionand migrane headaches,[11,12] primary dysmenorrhea,[13] mitral valve prolapse,[14] and sympathetic hypersensitivity.[15] muscle deconditioning and microtrauma,[16] muscle spasm and ischemia,[17] and sexual abuse.[18]

Dysfunction of the Nervous, Endocrine and Immune Systems

Immune system dysfunction either leading to or resulting from viral infections has been associated with chronic fatigue syndrome and fibromyalgia. Using advanced analytical techniques a defect in T-cell activation was found in fibromyalgia patients.[19] Research findings of immunologic dysfunction and neuroendocrine changes suggest the possible dysregulation of interactions between the nervous system and the immune system.[20]

Among the physiological imbalances observed in patients with fibromyalgia are immunologic dysfunction[21] including defects in T-cell activation,[22] possible viral injury to cellular calcium channels,[23] neuroendocrine dysregulation[24] including sleep disturbances,[25] and possible serotonin deficiency.[26] It has been postulated that the role of viral infection in fibromyalgia may involve viral damage to calcium channels in the cellular membrane.[27] Calcium is a critically involved in the cellular death process called apoptosis. Significant muscle abnormalities including Type-II fiber atrophy and a moth-eaten appearance in Type-I fibers are present in fibromyalgia.[28] Many have hypothesized that skeletal muscle is the "end organ" responsible for the pain of fibromyalgia[29] but it is becoming increasingly apparent that the nervous system, immune, and hormonal systems are intimately involved as well.[30]

Many researchers and clinicians believe that neurohormonal abnormalities are the root cause of FM and CFIDS.[31] The interconnectedness of the neural and hormonal systems certainly creates a challenging puzzle to sort out. Patients with FM exhibit disturbances of the major stress-response systems, the hypothalmic-pituitary-adrenal (HPA) axis, and the sympathetic nervous system. Many clinical features of FM and related disorders, such as widespread pain and fatigue, could in fact be related to the observed neurohormonal perturbations.[32]

Shifts in growth hormone (GH) and insulin-like growth factor-1 (IGF-1) have been a focus of intense research. Some studies have measured significant decreases in GH levels in FM patients,[33,34] while others have shown a normal balance of GH to IGF-1.[35,36] Still others have postulated that the low IGF-1 levels in patients with FM are a secondary phenomenon due to hypothalamic-pituitary-GH axis dysfunction.[37] Other studies point to acute cortisol release, or a drop in norepinephrine, which in turn induces low IGF-1 levels.[38] Sufficient benefit has been derived from at least one hormonal protocol to warrant the granting of a patent for the treatment of FM via hormonal manipulation.[39]

In any condition where metabolism and energy levels are involved the thyroid gland and the hormones it produces must be considered. The existence of low thyroid symptoms in fibromyalgia, in spite of the presence of normal thyroid hormone levels prompted Lowe, et al. to propose that a genetic defect may be the root cause of FM. Lowe proposed that a defect in the c-erbA-beta-1 gene or the c-erbA-alpha-1 gene would result in low-affinity thyroid-hormone receptors that prevent normal thyroid hormone regulation of transcription. Virtually every feature of fibromyalgia corresponds to signs or symptoms associated with failed transcription regulation by thyroid hormone.[40]

Biochemical Abnormalities

Many different biochemical imbalances are common in FM. These imbalances include diminished rates of glucose phosphorylation,[41] reduced erythrocyte magnesium (Mg) levels,[42] increased concentrations of homocysteine,[43] abnormal cellular carnitine metabolism,[44] mercury exposure,[45]

Need for a Holistic Approach

With so many correlations and contributing factors it is hard to determine which is the cause and which is the effect in analyzing fibromyalgia. It may also be the case that each of these factors may contribute slightly and in an additive manner resulting in overall poor performance and pain. Such an additive relationship may not be apparent especially when tests show that the individual parameters are all within the normal range albeit on the lower end of the range. This effect can be visually depicted as a spiral staircase with each step leading either up or down depending on whether the factor is improving or degrading thus leading to the proverbial "vicious cycle"[46] or its opposite, the "precious cycle."[47]

FOODS
Different people respond differently to the foods they eat. Some do better on a high carbohydrate diet some do better on a high protein diet. Because of the different response rates we

have to the different carbohydrate-fat-protein ratios of our diet it is best to investigate what your best food ratios are rather than follow whatever trend is currently popular. A self-scored questionnaire format has been developed and is available to those who wish to get some guidance in determining the proper food ratios for themselves as and individual.[48]

SUPPLEMENTS
Supplementation is important for all of us but it is especially critical for fibromyalgia sufferers. The section on Nutritional Supplementation goes through a detailed discussion of the various supplements that have been beneficial in relieving fibromyalgia.

EXERCISE
Dr. Joe Elrod's book *Reversing Fibromyalgia* details an exercise program specifically designed for improving both strength and flexibility.[49] Readers are referred to this text for specific exercise guidelines.

STRESS MANAGEMENT
A psychosomatic syndrome is defined as a syndrome in which psychological processes play a substantial role in the etiology of the illness in some of the patients.[50] The extent of the biological and psychosocial contributions vary among these syndromes as well as among individuals with the same syndrome. The phenomena of the somatoform disorders are caused by clustering of psychosomatic syndromes or their incomplete or atypical manifestations and a low sensation threshold.[51]

Psychiatric Diagnostic Interview data failed to discriminate in any major way between primary fibromyalgia syndrome and rheumatoid arthritis. These data do not support the psychopathology model as the primary explanation of the symptoms of primary fibromyalgia syndrome.[52] Other clinicians similarly have observed that pschological factors are detectable in only a low percentage of their fibromyalgia patients.[53] Nevertheless instruction in coping strategies in a structured pain school have been shown to be a useful addition to other treatments of fibromyalgia.[54] Family support is also a great advantage to fibromyalgia sufferers in their day-to-day struggles with pain and depression.[55] On the other hand emotionally traumatic events, such as sexual abuse, do not appear to be specific factors causing fibromyalgia, but they are correlated with the number and severity of associated symptoms.[56]

Personality Profiles

Many personality codings and classifications have been published. Many of these have used colors to code the various styles so as to avoid any inference of there being good and/or bad personalities.[57,58] Other systems have sought to align questionnaire responses to brain dominance. Left-brain dominance has been aligned with sequential thinking while right-brain dominance is associated with holistic thought patterns.[59] Herrmann refined the latter system to include a second dimension leading to a quadrant system of cerebral and limbic components.[60]

Each of these systems has strengths and weaknesses. Some of the weaknesses inherent in these systems results from the use of nebulous descriptors when defining the various dimensions of personality. A recently developed system utilizes a four quadrant personality characterization involving the four descriptors Life, Intuitive, Formal, and Expedient. The initial letters of these four words spells the word LIFE. An additional dimension involving past, present, and future perceptions and projections is incorporated in a second level refinement described as Core, Expected, and Desired tendencies. A written assessment tool can be obtained and processed for a nominal fee.[61]

One of the dangers associated with much of the pop-psychology of the last forty years has been a detachment from responsibility. Self-awareness and self-acceptance can only be truly successful if, coupled with the assertion of both our individual rights, there is an acceptance of our responsibilities for ourselves and to others.

Relaxation Techniques

Relaxation techniques can involve any and all aspects of the human experience. For some exercise is a great reliever. Others immerse themselves in music or service to others which both helps to relax and renew while putting into perspective the petty annoyances common to all lives. Some seek solitude others seek intense involvement. Each is worthwhile as means of connecting the individual to himself and his fellow beings.

SLEEP

An abnormal sleep pattern is a widely accepted cause for fibromyalgia.[62] A serotonin deficiency in the brain has been suggested to be of significance in fibromyalgia syndrome. Serotonin mediates both pain perception and non-REM sleep.[63] Nevertheless the standard use of tricyclic antidepressants[64] to modulate the sleep disorder has yielded less than excellent results.[65]

Regardless of the precise source of the hormonal contribution there is general agreement that disruption of the neuroendocrine axes may be one of the links between disturbed sleep and muscle pain.[66,67,68,69] Indeed, the discovery of the unstable early night sleep of FM patients reinforces the postulate that nighttime hormone (e.g., growth hormone) disturbance is an causative factor for FM.[70,71,72,73] The cascade of sleep deprivation, leading to hormone imbalance, muscle pain and fatigue, is further supported by sleep deprivation studies that created symptoms almost identical to FM.[74] What is clear is that sleep is essential to health and wellness, while the lack of restorative sleep contributes heavily to the burden of fibromyalgia.

ALTERNATE THERAPIES

It has been reported that ninety-eight percent of fibromyalgia sufferers used at least one complementary treatment strategy over the preceding 6 months.[75,76] Most of this interest in complementary therapies was seen to be generated by poor clinical results using conventional medical protocols.[77] Acupuncture was reported to be a good additional method to relieve or to eliminate pain in fibromyalgia patients.[78]

SUMMARY

In a review of rehabilitation approaches for fibromyalgia, D. Rosen stated: "Although treatment always starts at the tissue level, a good treatment programme must always be holistic in nature and treat the tissues, the patient as a whole, and his or her environmental stressors and contingencies as well....the major goal of all treatment programmes is to restore individuals to functional lifestyles and to promote both physical and emotional flexibility, balance and 'wellness'."[79]

Nutritional Support

TRANSFER FACTOR

Our health and quality of life are directly influenced by our immune system. Today many factors contribute to the general weakening of our bodies' defenses. Antibiotics, commonly viewed as the most important advance in the history of medicine, have begun to fail as more and more microbes develop resistant strains. Fortunately recent research has uncovered a natural agent which can potentially save lives and increase the quality of life for many people.

Transfer Factors are small immune messenger molecules that are produced by all higher organisms.[80,81] They are both regulators of the immune system and carriers of the essential information needed by the immune system to identify foreign organisms. Transfer factors are unique to the infectious agent but are not dependent on the individual that produced them. Transfer factors produced by one person can be used in another person without concern for blood type or any other difference. In fact transfer factors produced in animals and man are the same.

Colostrum, the first milk that a mother provides her offspring immediately after birth, is a rich source of transfer factors. This is nature's way of quickly educating a niave infant in the hazards of a microbe infested world. The abundant source for transfer factors is found in the colostrum produced by cattle. Unfortunately many people are allergic to milk proteins or are lactose intolerant making whole colostrum an unfit source of transfer factors for these persons. Recent technological breakthroughs have solved this problem. Transfer factors can now be efficiently isolated from bovine colostrum.

Transfer factor preparations have been used to educate the immune systems of persons suffering from chronic fatigue syndrome, a condition almost identical to fibromyalgia. Chronic fatigue, like fibromyalgia, is a syndrome with multiple contributing factors not the least of which is persistent viral infection.[82] Because of the multiple infectious agents that can contribute to chronic fatigue syndrome, poly-valent (reactivity to more than one organism) transfer factor preparations have been used.[83] Success was reported in 35 out of 39.[84]

Another pilot study used poly-valent transfer factors with known potency for Epstein Barr and Cytomegalovirus . In this study two of the fourteen patients demonstrated total remission, while seven of the fourteen showed marked improvement. Use of a non-specific transfer factor provided marked improvement in three out of six patients.[85]

Immunological dysfunction is not the only contributing factor in fibromylagia but it is a critical issue that must be addressed. The involvement of viral infections in a large percentage of fibromyalgia cases has led researchers to propose viral infections as the initiating event for many fibromyalgia suffers.[86] Overcoming the residual effects of viral damage and elimination of the persistant viral infections may be key to the recovery from fibromyalgia.

MAGNESIUM

The role of magnesium in the treatment of fibromyalgia was first reported by Dr. G. E. Abraham's group in 1992.[87] Dr. Abraham's earlier gynecological work had demonstrated that dysmenorrhea[88] and PMS symptoms[89] were strongly correlated with deficient magnesium levels. Since 80 percent of the fibromyalgia suffers are women and the fact that there is a correlation between fibromyalgia and PMS one can reasonably assume that Dr. Abraham had seen some crossover benefits during his magnesium-PMS trials. In a later controlled study, Abraham, et al. confirmed this preliminary finding and demonstrated that significant reductions in pain/tenderness severity could be achieved during extended treatment with high doses of magnesium and malic acid (600 mg/day and 2400 mg/day respectively). No limiting risk factors were found.[90] Other researchers have found that fibromyalgia patients do indeed have significantly lower red blood cell magnesium levels compared to reference laboratory and osteoarthritis controls.[91] Reduced erythrocyte magnesium (Mg) levels have been reported in fibromyalgia syndrome (FS), chronic fatigue syndrome (CFS), myofascial pain syndrome (MPS), eosinophilia myalgia syndrome (EMS), and in patients with systemic lupus erythematosus (SLE).[92] These disorders have chronic pain as a common symptom. Low tissue levels of magnesium in fibromyalgia were confirmed by Clauw[93] who also showed that low muscular magnesium levels correlated with low pain tolerance.[94] Similar magnesium deficiencies were also found in patients with eosinophilia-myalgia syndrome.[95]

Magnesium deficiencies are also associated with neuronal/emotional disorders as illustrated by the following findings. Magnesium levels in cerebrospinal fluid (CSF) were lowered in depressed people, signaling potentially low levels of magnesium in the.[96] Magnesium deficiencies in humans have been linked with symptoms of depression, agitation, and disorientation.[97] Low mitochondrial magnesium levels are thought to contribute to the triggering of migraines.[98]

Calcium channel blocking agents are widely used cardiovascular drugs. It is well established that the most effective natural calcium channel blocker is magnesium.[99] A deficiency in magnesium has been identified as the primary causative factor in "generalized cardiovascular-metabolic disease(s)" known as "Syndrome X."[100] Magnesium has been called the premier cardiovascular mineral.[101] Knowing the importance of magnesium to heart muscle, it should not be surprising that magnesium would also be important in the generalized muscular dysfunction seen in fibromyalgia.

Why is magnesium so important? Magnesium is involved with every major energy production and transport function in the body![102] Because of this magnesium supplementation has beneficial impacts on fatigue and pain. Pain is a neuro-physical factor designed to limit activity and thus limit excessive energy demand and the cellular damage that occurs when insufficient energy is available to meet the demands.

B-VITAMINS

Cellular magnesium abnormalities have been shown to be associated with faulty thiamin metabolism.[103] Thiamin, and essential vitamin, is a critical cofactor in cellular energy production and transport.

All fibromyalgia and chronic fatigue syndrome patients tested were found to have elevated homocysteine levels in their central nervous systems.[104] Homocysteine has been identified as a high risk factor in cardiovascular disease as well.[105] High homocysteine levels were correlated with low levels of vitamin B12 and high levels of fatiguability.[106] It is known that vitamin B12 deficiency causes a deficient remethylation of homocysteine.[107]

MALIC ACID

The role of malic acid is postulated to involve the enhanced formation of NADH and oxaloacetate by the action of the citric acid cycle. The citric acid cycle, sometimes called the tricarboxylic acid cycle or the Krebs cycle, is the main energy producing cycle of the body. Malic acid enters the citric acid cycle at the most efficient site and is quickly converted into NADH and subsequently into useable energy in the form of three ATP.[108] ATP acts as a battery, storing energy while it is being transported from the mitochondrial power plant to the various enzymatic factories of the cell where it is consumed. Magnesium plays a critical role in the stabilization of ATP. Without magnesium ATP is made but falls apart before it can be delivered to the enzymatic factories. This leads not only to inefficient and weak cells but also to cellular damage when the energy carried by the NADH or ATP is randomly released in an uncontrolled fashion. It is important to note that both NADH and oxaloacetate that are formed from malic acid metabolism are important cellular factors in their own right. An additional role for malic acid may be as a chelator for alumium as discussed by Abraham and Flechas.[109]

GLUCOSAMINE AND CARTILAGE

The musculoskeletal system is comprised of the muscles, the bones, and the joints. Fibromyalgia is often called a soft tissue arthritis, while osteoarthritis and rheumatoid arthritis involve the joints. One of the cross-over problems with either joint or muscular pain is the likelihood that problems in one part of the musculoskeletal system often result in excessive strain on the other parts of the system. For example joint pain can lead to a favored gait that puts a repetitive abnormal stress on muscles resulting in muscle strain, injury and pain. Treating one part of the system without regard for the other components of the system is a hit-or-miss approach.

The use of glucosamine and and cartilage hydrolysates in the nutritional treatment of arthritic conditions has been well documented in two books by Dr. Luke Bucchi.[110,111] Glucosamine accelerates the repair of tissue injuries[112] and cartilage preparations exerted a protective affect on the heart.[113] These soft tissue affects are in addition to the documented benefits of glucosamine and cartilage hydrolysates on joint function and pain reduction. The availability of glucosamine limits the body's ability to make glucosaminylglycans (GAGs) the main component of the synovial fluid that greases our joints.[114] Cartilage hydrolysates and the chondrotin sulfates they contain protect the GAGs from being degraded. In addition cartilage preparations have been shown to reduce dementia by improving blood flow and most likely oxygen delivery.[115] Low oxygen availability is known as hypoxia and is thought to contribute to muscle dysfunction in fibromyalgia. Glucosamine improves inflamatory conditions as well as acting as a free-radical scavaenger.

METHYLSULFONYLMETHANE (MSM)
Methylsulfonylmethane (MSM) is a nutritional food supplement found in all foods—milk, fruits, meats and vegetables. MSM has been well studied by Dr. Stanley Jacobs. Dr. Jacobs clinical trials have demonstrated the safety and benefits of MSM as a source of organic sulfur.[116] Methylsulfonylmethane (MSM) has demonstrated the remarkable ability to reduce muscle soreness, and cramps. MSM also helps alleviate the pain associated with systemic inflammatory disorders. The observations that allergies are also reduced may further suggest an interaction with the immune system.[117]

BOSWELLIA SERRATA
Boswellia serrata is a traditional Ayurvedic treatment for joint pain and inflamation. In ancient times this material was known as frankinscence.[118,119] The traditionally established safety of boswellia serrata has recently been reinforced by modern pharmacological studies.[120] Boswellia serrata was found to have slow-acting long term anti-inflammatory affects.[121,122] These anti-inflammatory affects are beneficial to those suffering from adjuvant induced arthritis.[123] Mechanistically, Boswellia serrata appears to function as a natural inhibitor of leukotriene biosynthesis.[124] .

CYSTEINE AND DERIVATIVES
The combination of abnormally low plasma cystine and glutamine levels, low natural killer (NK) cell activity, skeletal muscle wasting or muscle fatigue, and increased rates of urea production defines a complex of abnormalities that Droege and coworkers

have labeled "low CG syndrome."[125] The symptoms associated with "low CG syndrome" are common features in a number of seemingly unrelated conditions including chronic fatigue syndrome, fibromyalgia, HIV infection, cancer, major injuries, sepsis, Crohn's disease, ulcerative colitis, and to some extent in overtrained athletes and old age.

Cysteine plays a critical role in the prevention of skeletal muscle wasting and fatigue conditions. The interrelated role of the immune system with cachexia (wasting) was further illustrated by the discovery of the triggering effects of Interleukin-6 (IL-6) which are sustained by an abnormal cysteine metabolism.[126]

The loss of body cell mass (wasting) is correlated with low baseline levels of plasma glutamine, arginine, and cystine. Wasting in healthy individuals appears to be self-terminating as glutamine, arginine, and cystine are adjusted to higher levels that stabilize body cell mass. Since cysteine and glutamine are related, the regulatory role of cysteine was tested in subjects with relatively low glutamine levels. Supplementation with N-acetyl-cysteine increased the ratio of body cell mass to body fat. This indicates that cysteine does play a regulatory role in the maintenance of healthy body cell mass. In contrast the placebo group showed a loss of body cell mass and an increase in body fat, suggesting that body protein had been converted into other forms of chemical energy.[127] It is not surprising therefore that N-acetylcysteine pretreatment improved human muscle performance during fatiguing exercise.[128]

Sepsis, a toxic infectious condition, also results in muscle wasting. The requirement for cysteine in the maintenance of acid balance inside the cell is often sacrificed in this condition as cysteine is used for protein synthesis and antioxidant (glutathione) production.[129] Cystiene supplementation is recommended during times of sepsis.

The increased but unmet magnesium and cysteine requirements of fibromyalgia sufferers may explain the muscle pain they experience.

GLUTAMINE AND UREA

Plasma cystine levels regulate nitrogen balance and body cell mass. The importance of maintaining normal cystine levels is so critical that skeletal muscle protein is cannibalized in order to supply the increased cystine demand.[130] In the short term this may be useful but in chronic conditions it is very damaging as it leads to an excess production of urea at the expense of glutamine which is needed for the fueling of the immune system.

GLUTATHIONE

The altered redox state in patients with RA indicate an important role for N-acetyl-L-cysteine (NAC) in the restoring of glutathione (GSH) levels in hyporesponsive joint T cells.[131,132] Such repletions of glutathione with NAC are well established.[133]

GENERAL ANTIOXIDANT

Cysteine and N-acetyl-L-cysteine (NAC) are good antioxidants in their own right separate from their role as glutathione precursors. Some of the conditions in which cysteine and NAC are important include ulcerative colitis,[134] lens damage from low level radiation,135 and rheumatoid arthritis.[136,137]

CREATINE

A patent has been issued for the use of certain creatine preparations for treatment of fibromyalgia and other types of myopathy and cachectic states.[138]

Hormonal Supplementation and Herbal Calmatives

MELATONIN

Melatonin is a hormone whose natural daily cyclic variation assists us in attaining deep levels of sleep. As we get older our ability to produce melatonin drops significantly and may play a major role in aging and its related declines in functional efficiency.[139]

Melatonin regulates the sleep-wake cycle by inhibiting the mechanism used by the central nervous system to generate wakefulness.[140] Administration of melatonin effects the three main characteristics of human sleep: 1) latency to sleep onset, 2)sleep consolidation "slow waves" and "sleep spindles," and 3) REM sleep.[141] It has been predicted that in the near future melatonin administration will become as useful as bright light exposure in the treatment of circadian phase disorders.[142] The sleep-promoting effects of melatonin typically are observed within one hour following treatment, regardless of the time melatonin is administered.[143] For this reason it is advisable to restrict melatonin ingestion to the time just before retiring for the evening.

GRIFFONIA SIMPLICIFOLIA, NATURAL SOURCE OF 5-HYDROXYTRYPTOPHAN (5-HTP)

The high prevalence of migraines in the population of fibromyalgia sufferers suggests a common ground shared by fibromyalgia and migraine. Migraines are characterized by a defect in the serotonergic and adrenergic systems. A parallel dramatic failure of serotonergic systems and a defect of adrenergic transmission have been evidenced to affect fibromyalgia sufferers, too. Enhancing serotonergic analgesia while increasing adrenergically mediated analgesia seems to be an important tool in fibromyalgia.[144] The administration of 5-hydroxytryptophan (5-HTP) significantly improved fibromyalgia.[145] All the clinical variables (number of tender points, anxiety, pain intensity, quality of sleep, fatigue) showed a significant improvement when patients were given 5-HTP during extended treatment periods.[146,147]

PREGNENOLONE

Receptor-active neurosteroids may represent an important class of neuromodulators that can rapidly alter central nervous system excitability via novel nongenomic mechanisms.[148] Pregnenolone is one of the critical neurosteroids and has the ability to modify the sleep EEG in humans, which suggests its potential benefit as a memory enhancer.[149,150] Studies conducted on acute shook stress indicate that there is a relationship between neurosteroid levels and the functional and emotional state of the stressed animals.[151] A shift in the metabolism of pregnenolone may be necessary for survival during chronic severe stress.[152] Unfortunately, in chronic diseases there is an observed drop in pregnenolone levels.[153] Mercury poisoning causes a defect in the conversion of cholesterol to pregnenolone, which accounts in part for the diminished stress tolerance.[154] In animal studies pregnenolone significantly reduced exploratory anxiety.[155] A very low dose of pregnenolone significantly increases slow-wave, deep sleep in healthy males.[156]

ST JOHN'S WORT

Numerous studies on St. John's wort extracts[157] involving depressed patients have been published in the last 20 years. A total of 12 placebo-controlled trials with hypericum extracts were performed, yielding mostly positive results. In Germany, St. John's wort extracts are among the most widely prescribed antidepressants as well as the best selling, non-prescription antidepressant in the country.[158] St John's wort extracts have consistently matched the antidepressant efficacy of synthetic antidepressants such as amitriptyline, imipramine, and maprotiline. On the other hand, the tolerability of St John's wort extract was clearly superior to imipramine[159] and amitriptyline.[160] Researchers observed beneficial effects within two weeks.

Seasonal affective disorder (SAD) is a subgroup of major depression. St. John's wort extracts, light therapy (LT), and specific antidepressants have been shown to be beneficial. When bright light therapy combined with St. John's wort extract was compared to St. John's wort extract alone, no significant difference indicated that the benefit was coming from the extract itself. St. John's wort extract was well tolerated and was recommended as a potentially efficient therapy in patients with SAD.[161]

KAVA

Another herbal extract used for its calming effects on people with anxiety disorders is kava-kava, which in some cases is recommended over synthetic psychopharmacological agents.[162] Three randomized placebo-controlled double-blind trials on anxiety disorders have recently been completed.[163,164,165] In each clinical study, treatment demonstrated a high level of efficacy of kava extract associated with very good tolerance of the preparation. A good multidisciplinary overview of kava-kava is available for those who desired further detailed information.[166]

Stages and Recovery

INTENSITY OF CONDITION

Fibromyalgia develops and is overcome in stages. Only the most severe stages are recognized as the condition we call fibromyalgia. The more severe stages may require greater nutritional and emotional support while only a mild exercise program may be possible. When partial recovery has been achieved a more balanced program of nutrition stress management and exercise should be possible.

Most of us would agree that muscle pain is a common feature of many people's lives. About 11 percent of the general population suffer from chronic widespread pain. This primary symptom of fibromyalgia is much more common than previously assumed. Those suffer with chronic widespread pain were also found to more likely report symptoms of fatigue and depression.[167] Insomnia has also been listed as one of the most common health disorders in America. It may be more honest for us to claim normal poor health than for us to claim normal good health.

TIME AND PATIENCE

Fibromyalgia is not a trivial syndrome. A holistic approach is most effective in dealing with the multiple contributing factors of fibromyalgia. It also takes time and patience to overcome this condition.

PRECIOUS CYCLES AND VICIOUS CYCLES

Any action that we take that harms us starts us on a vicious cycle downward. Similarly any action that we take that builds and benefits us starts us on an upward spiral called a precious cycle. The information in this booklet is designed to guide you to those actions that will lead you to an upward precious cycle. Health after all is the most precious physical, emotional, mental and spiritual wealth we can ever possess.

Summary

Chronic conditions like fibromyalgia are difficult to manage and frustrating for both the patient and the care-giver. But when patience can be applied and confidence achieved, a positive relationship can result and the patient can be helped.[168]

Knowing exactly which of the multiple causative factors may be present in your fibromyalgia condition may be helpful and even comforting. Putting a face on our fears brings them to a manageable size. Identifying the source of our pain helps us focus our energies constructively. It is increasingly apparent, however, that there is not likely to be any one factor that is affecting us but rather a multitude of small contributions. None of these are necessarily significant by themselves, but taken together they can be a tremendous burden. Through a comprehensive, holistic program of diet, exercise, stress management including adequate deep refreshing sleep, and supplementation, small additive changes can culminate in an optimal personal wellness.

We hope that those of you who suffer from fibromyalgia or know someone who sufferes from fibromyalgia will be able to take courage and obtain hope from the information we have discussed above. Fibromyalgia is real and there are real solutions. Finding the approach that will most closely match your personality and individual metabolism are key to recovering from fibromyalgia and going on to leading a more rich and fulfilling life.

Notes

1. Fibromyalgia The Copenhagen Declaration. Quintner J. Lancet (N Am Ed) 1992, 340(8827), 1103.
2. The fibromyalgia syndrome: musculoskeletal pathophysiology. Geel SE. Semin Arthritis Rheum 1994, 23(5), 347-53
3. Fibromyalgia—a clinical entity? Henriksson KG, Bengtsson A. Can J Physiol Pharmacol 1991, 69(5), 672-7.
4. Fibromyalgia—a clinical entity? Henriksson KG, Bengtsson A. Can J Physiol Pharmacol 1991, 69(5), 672-7.
5. Fibromyalgia and chronic fatigue syndrome: Similarities and differences. Buchwald D. Rheumatic Disease Clinics of North America 1996, 22(2), 219-243.
6. The relationship between fibromyalgia and major depressive disorder. Hudson JI, Pope HG Jr. Rheumatic Disease Clinics of North America 1996, 22(2), 285-303.
7. Fibromyalgia, chronic fatigue syndrome, and myofascial pain syndrome. Goldenberg DL. Current Opinion in Rheumatology 1995, 7(2), 127-135.
8. Chronic fatigue syndrome and a disorder resembling Sj.ogren's syndrome: preliminary report. Calabrese L H, Davis M E, Wilke W S, Clin Infect Dis 1994, 18(Suppl 1), S28-31.
9. Bowel sysfunction and irritable bowel syndrome in fibromyalgia patients. Sivri A, Cindas A, Dincer F, Sivri B. Clin Rheumatol 1996, 15(3), 283-6.
10. The pathogenesis of chronic pain and fatigue syndromes, with special reference to fibromyalgia. Clauw DJ. Medical Hypotheses 1995, 44, 369-378.
11. Primary fibromyalgia syndrome and myofacial pain syndrome: Clinical features and muscel pathology. Yunus MB, Raman KIUP, Raman, KK. Arch Phys Med Rehabil 1988, 69, 451-4.
12. Fibromyalgia and migraine, two faces of the same mechanism. Serotonin as the common clue for pathogenesis and therapy. Nicolodi M., Sicuteri F. Adv Exp Med Biol 1996, 398, 373-9.
13. Primary fibromyalgia syndrome and myofacial pain syndrome: Clinical features and muscel pathology. Yunus MB, Raman KIUP, Raman, KK. Arch Phys Med Rehabil 1988, 69, 451-4.
14. Prevalance of mitral valve prolapse in primary fibromyalgia: a pilot investigation. Pellegrino MJ, Van Fossen D, Gordon C, Ryan JM, Waylonis GW. Arch Phys Med Rehabil 1989, 70, 541-3.
15. An investigation of sympathetic hypersensitivity in chronic fatigue syndrome. Sendrowski DP, Buker EA, Gee SS. Optom Vis Sci 1997, 74(8), 660-3.
16. Beyond fibromyalgia: ideas on etiology and treatment. Bennett RM. J Rheumatol Suppl 1989, 19, 185-91.
17. Muscle pathology in primary fibromyalgia syndrome: a light microscopic, histochemical and ultrastructural study. Kalyan-Raman UP, Kalyan-Raman K, Yunus MB, Masi AT. J Rheumatol 1984, 11(6), 808-13.
18. The prevalence of sexual abuse in women with fibromyalgia. Taylor ML, Trotter DR, Csuka ME. Arthritis Rheum 1995, 38(2), 229-34.
19. Lymphocyte subpopulations in patients with primary fibromyalgia. Hernanz W, Valenzuela A, Quijada J, Garcia A, de la Iglesia JL, Gutierrez A, Povedano J, Moreno I, Sanchez B. J Rheumatol 1994, 21(11), 2122-4.
20. Chronic fatigue syndrome. 1: Etiology and pathogenesis. Farrar DJ, Locke SE, Kantrowitz FG. Behav Med 1995, 21(1), 5-16.
21. Chronic fatigue syndrome. 1: Etiology and pathogenesis. Farrar DJ, Locke SE, Kantrowitz FG. Behav Med 1995, 21(1), 5-16.
22. Lymphocyte subpopulations in patients with primary fibromyalgia. Hernanz W, Valenzuela A, Quijada J, Garcia A, de la Iglesia JL, Gutierrez A, Povedano J, Moreno I, Sanchez B. J Rheumatol 1994, 21(11), 2122-4.
23. The etiology and possible treatment of chronic fatigue syndrome/fibromyalgia. Lund-Olesen

LH, Lund-Olesen K. Med Hypotheses 1994, 43(1), 55-8.
24. Chronic fatigue syndrome. 1: Etiology and pathogenesis. Farrar DJ, Locke SE, Kantrowitz FG. Behav Med 1995, 21(1), 5-16.
25. Sleep disturbances, fibromyalgia and primary Sj.ogren's syndrome. Tishler M, Barak Y, Paran D, Yaron M. Clin Exp Rheumatol 1997, 15(1), 71-4.
26. Fibromyalgia] Siegmeth W, Geringer EM. Wien Med Wochenschr 1995, 145(14), 320-5,
27. The etiology and possible treatment of chronic fatigue syndrome/fibromyalgia. Lund-Olesen LH, Lund-Olesen K. Med Hypotheses 1994, 43(1), 55-8.
28. Muscle pathology in primary fibromyalgia syndrome: a light microscopic, histochemical and ultrastructural study. Kalyan-Raman UP, Kalyan-Raman K, Yunus MB, Masi AT. J Rheumatol 1984, 11(6), 808-13.
29. Beyond fibromyalgia: ideas on etiology and treatment. Bennett RM. J Rheumatol Suppl 1989, 19, 185-91.
30. Fibromyalgia. A neuro-immuno-endocrinologic syndrome? Olin R. Lakartidningen 1995, 92(8), 755-8, 761-3.
31. Evidence that abnormalities of central neurohormonal systems are key to understanding fibromyalgia and chronic fatigue syndrome. Crofford LJ, Demitrack MA. Rheumatic Disease Clinics of North America 1996, 22(2), 267-284.
32. Neurohormonal perturbations in fibromyalgia. Crofford LJ, Engleberg NC, Demitrack MA. Baillieres Clin Rheumatol 1996,10(2), 365-78.
33. Low growth hormone secretion in patients with fibromyalgia: A preliminary report on 10 patients and 10 controls. Bagge E, Bengtsson B-A, Carlsson L, Carlsson J. J Rheumatol 1998, 25(1), 145-148.
34. Pituitary release of growth hormone and prolactin in the primary fibromyalgia syndrome. Griep EN, Boersma JW, de Kloet ER. J Rheumatol 1994, 21(11), 2125-30.
35. Insulin-like growth factor-I (Somatomedin C) levels in chronic fatigue syndrome and fibromyalgia. Buchwald D, Umali J, Stene M. J Rheumatol 1996, 23(4), 739-742.
36. A controlled study on serum insulin-like growth factor-I and urinary excretion of growth hormone in fibromyalgia. Jacobsen S, Main K, Danneskiold-Samsoe B, Skakkebaek NE. J Rheumatol 1995, 22(6), 1138-40.
37. Hypothalamic-pituitary-insulin-like growth factor-I axis dysfunction in patients with fibromyalgia. Bennett, R. M.; Cook, D. M.; Clark, S. R.; Burckhardt, C. S.; Campbell, S. M. J Rheumatol 1997, 24(7), 1384-9.
38. Somatomedin C (insulin-like growth factor 1) levels decrease during acute changes of stress related hormones. Relevance for fibromyalgia. Ferraccioli G, Guerra, P, Rizzi V, Baraldo M, Salaffi F, Furlanut M, Bartoli E. J Rheumatol 1994, 21(7), 1332-4.
39. Therapeutic treatment of fibromyalgia- Bennett, RM. USP 05378686, 1995-01-03.
40. Mutations in the c-erbA-beta-1 gene: Do they underlie euthyroid fibromyalgia? Lowe JC, Cullum ME, Graf LH, Jr, Yellin J. Medical Hypotheses 1997, 48(2), 125-135.
41. [Determination of regional rate of glucose metabolism in lumbar muscles in patients with generalized tendomyopathy using dynamic 18F-FDG PET.] Frey LD, Locher JT, Hrycaj P, Stratz T, Kovac C, Mennet P, Muller W. Z Rheumatol 1992, 51(5), 238-42.
42. Magnesium deficiency in systemic lupus erythematosus. Romano TJ. J Nutritional & Environmental Medicine (Abingdon) 1997, 7(2), 107-111.
43. Increased concentrations of homocysteine in the cerebrospinal fluid inpatients with fibromyalgia and chronic fatigue syndrome. Regland B, Andersson M, Abrahamsson L, Bagby J, Dyrehag LE, Gottfries CG. Scand J Rheumatol 26(41997), 301-307.
44. Abnormal cellular carnitine metabolism in chronic fatigue syndrome. Kuratsune H, Yamaguti K, Takahashi M, Tagawa S, Machii T, Kitani T. EOS-Rivista di Immunologia ed Immunofarmacologia 1995, 15(1-2), 40-44.
45. Mercury exposure from dental amalgam fillings in the etiology of primary fibromyalgia: a pilot study [letter]. Kotter I, Durk H, Saal JG, Kroiher A, Schweinsberg F. J Rheumatol 1995, 22(11), 2194-5.

46. [Does fibromyalgia exist?] Serratrice G. Rev Rhum Mal Osteoartic 1990, 57(3, Pt 2), 260-6.
47. Private communication from David Lisonbee.
48. To obtain a copy of the foods assessment questionaire, call 4-Life ResearchTM at 1-888-4-Life-74 (1-888-454-3374) and request a copy of the Instant Biosignature.TM
49. Reversing Fibromyalgia. Elrod J. Woodland Books Publishers. Pleasant Grove, UT 1997.
50. Psychosomatic syndromes, somatization and somatoform disorders [see comments]. Kellner R. Psychother Psychosom 1994, 61(1-2), 4-24. Comment in:, Psychother Psychosom, 1994, 61(1-2), 1-3.
51. Psychosomatic syndromes, somatization and somatoform disorders [see comments]. Kellner R. Psychother Psychosom 1994, 61(1-2), 4-24. Comment in:, Psychother Psychosom, 1994, 61(1-2), 1-3.
52. Psychiatric status of patients with primary fibromyalgia, patients with rheumatoid arthritis, and subjects without pain: a blind comparison of DSM-III diagnoses. Ahles TA, Khan SA, Yunus MB, Spiegel DA, Masi AT. Am J Psychiatry 1991, 148(12), 1721-6.
53. [Does fibromyalgia exist?] Serratrice G. Rev Rhum Mal Osteoartic 1990, 57(3, Pt 2), 260-6.
54. Patients with fibromyalgia in pain school. Kogstad O, Hintringer F. J Musculoskel Pain 1993, 1(3-4), 261-266.
55. The contribution of family cohesion and the pain-coping process to depressive symptoms in fibromyalgia. Nicassio PM, Radojevic V, Schoenfield-Smith K, Dwyer K. Ann Behav Med 1995, 17(4), 349-356.
56. The prevalence of sexual abuse in women with fibromyalgia. Taylor ML, Trotter DR, Csuka ME. Arthritis Rheum 1995, 38(2), 229-34.
57. Life Colors. Oslie P. New World Library, San Rafael, CA 1991.
58. The Color Code. Hartman TD. Taylor Don Hartman Publishers, Trabuco Canyon, CA 1987.
59. Left Brain, Right Brain. Springer SP, Deutsch G. WH Freeman Publishers, New York, NY 1985.
60. The Creative Brain; Parts I and II. Herrmann N. Training and Development Journal, American Society for Training and Development, Washington D. C.
61. To obtain the assesment form and arrange for processing contact 4-Life Research at 1-888-4-LIFE-74 (1-888-454-3374) and request the complete BiosignatureTM form.
62. Sleep disturbances, fibromyalgia and primary Sj.ogren's syndrome. Tishler M, Barak Y, Paran D, Yaron M. Clin Exp Rheumatol 1997, 15(1), 71-4.
63. [Fibromyalgia.] Siegmeth W, Geringer EM. Wien Med Wochenschr 1995, 145(14), 320-5.
64. Tricyclic antidepressants in the treatment of insomnia. Ware JC. J Clin Psychiatry 1983, 44(9, Pt 2), 25-8.
65. Fibromyalgia. Part I. Review of the literature. Harvey CK, Cadena R, Dunlap L. J Am Podiatr Med Assoc 1993, 83(7), 412-5.
66. Fibromyalgia and the facts. Sense or nonsense. Bennett RM. Rheum Dis Clin North Am 1993, 19(1), 45-59.
67. Low levels of somatomedin C in patients with the fibromyalgia syndrome. A possible link between sleep and muscle pain. Bennett RM, Clark SR, Campbell SM, Burckhardt CS. Arthritis Rheum 1992, 35(10), 1113-6.
68. Therapeutic treatment of fibromyalgia- Bennett, RM. USP 05378686, 1995-01-03.
69. The origin of myopain: An integrated hypothesis of focal muscle changes and sleep disturbance in patients with the fibromyalgia syndrome. Bennett RM. J Musculoskel Pain 1993, 1(3-4), 95-112.
70. Low growth hormone secretion in patients with fibromyalgia: A preliminary report on 10 patients and 10 controls. Bagge E, Bengtsson B-A, Carlsson L, Carlsson J. J Rheumatol 1998, 25(1), 145-148.
71. Sleep, psychological distress, and stress arousal in women with fibromyalgia. Shaver JL, Lentz M, Landis CA, Heitkemper MM, Buchwald DS, Woods NF. Res Nurs Health 1997, 20(3), 247-57.
72. A controlled study on serum insulin-like growth factor-I and urinary excretion of growth hor-

mone in fibromyalgia. Jacobsen S, Main K, Danneskiold-Samsoe B, Skakkebaek NE. J Rheumatol 1995, 22(6), 1138-40.

73. Studies of sleep in fibromyalgia; techniques, clinical significance and future directions. Smythe HA. Brit J Rheum 1995, 34, 897-900. And references therein.

74. Induction of neurasthenic musculskeletal pain syndrome by selective sleep stage deprivation. Moldofsky H, Scarisbrick P. Psycosom Med 1976, 38, 35-44.

75. Psychosocial factors associated with complementary treatment use in fibromyalgia. Nicassio PM, Schuman C, Kim J, Cordova A, Weisman MH. J Rheumatol. 1997, 24 (10) 2008-13.

76. Alternative medicine use in fibromyalgia syndrone. Pioro-Boisset M, Esdaile JM, Fitzcharles MA. Arthritis Care Res. 1996, 9(1), 13-7.

77. [Guidelines for social medicine assessment and evaluation of primary fibromyalgia]

78. Efficiency of acupuncture in patients with fibromyalgia. Sprott H, Mueller W. Reumatologia (Warsaw) 1994, 32(4) 414-421.

79. Physical medicine and rehabilitation approaches to the management of myofascial pain and fibromyalgia syndromes. Rosen NB. Baillieres Clin Rheumatol 1994, 8(4) 881-916.

80. Transfer Factor: Natural immune booster. Hennen WJ. Woodland Publishers, Pleasant Grove, UT 1998.

81. Immunology, Immunopathology and Immunity. Sell S. Appleton and Lange: Stamford CT 1996.

82. Lessons from a piolot study on transfer factor in chronic fatigue syndrome. De Vinci C, Levine PH, Pizza G, Fudenberg HH, Orens P, Pearson G, Viza D. Biotherapy 1996, 9(1-3), 87-90.

83. The use of transfer factors in chronic fatigue syndrome: prospects and problems. Levine PH. Biotherapy 1996, 9(1-3), 77-9.

84. Transfer factor 1993: New frontiers. Fudenberg HH, Pizza G. Progress in Drug Res 1994 42, 309-400.

85. Lessons from a pilot study of transfer factor in chronic fatigue syndrome. De Vinci C, Levine PH, Pizza G, Fudenberg HH, Orens P, Pearson G, Viza D. Biotherapy 1996, 9(1-3), 87-90.

86. The etiology and possible treatment of chronic fatigue syndrome/fibromyalgia. Lund-Olesen LH, Lund-Olesen K. Med Hypotheses 1994, 43(1), 55-8.

87. Management of fibromyalgia: rationale for the use of magnesium and malic acid. Abraham, G. E.; Flechas, J. D. Journal of nutritional medicine 1992, 3 (1), 49-59.

88. Primary dysmenorrhea. Abraham, G. E. Clin Obstet Gynecol 1978, 21(1), 139-45.

89. a) Serum and red cell magnesium levels in patients with premenstrual tension. Abraham GE, Lubran MM. Am J Clin Nutr 1981, 34(11), 2364-6.

b) Primary dysmenorrhea. Abraham GE. Clin Obstet Gynecol 1978, 21(1), 139-45.

c) Nutritional factors in the etiology of the premenstrual tension syndromes. Abraham GE. J Reprod Med 1983, 28(7), 446-64.

d) Effect of vitamin B-6 on plasma and red blood cell magnesium levels in premenopausal women. Abraham GE, Schwartz UD, Lubran MM. Ann Clin Lab Sci 1981, 11(4), 333-6.

90. Treatment of fibromyalgia syndrome with Super Malic: a randomized,double blind, placebo controlled, crossover pilot study. Russell IJ, Michalek JE, Flechas JD, Abraham GE J Rheumatol 1995, 22(5), 953-8.

91. Magnesium deficiency in fibromyalgia syndrome. Romano TJ, Stiller JW J Nutritional Med 1994, 4(2) 165-167.

92. Magnesium deficiency in systemic lupus erythematosus. Romano TJ. J Nutritional & Environmental Med (Abingdon) 1997, 7(2) 107-111.

93. Low tissue levels of magnesium in fibromyalgia. Clauw DJ, Wilson B, Phadia S, Radulovic D, Katz P. Clinical Research 1994, 42(2), 141A.

94. Muscle intracellular magnesium levels correlate with pain tolerance infibromyalgia. Clauw D, Katz KWP, Rajan S. Arthritis & Rheumatism 1994, 37(9) S213.

95. Magnesium deficiency in the eosinophilia-myalgia syndrome. Report of clinical and bio-

chemical improvement with repletion. Clauw DJ, Wark K, Wilson B, Katz P, Rajan SS. Arthritis & Rheum 1994, 37(9), 1331-1334.

96. Cerebrospinal fluid magnesioum and calcium related to amine metabolites, diagnosis, and suicide attempts. Bancki CM, et al. Biol Psychiatry 1985, 20, 163-171.

97. Magnesium deficiency in chronic schizophrenia. Kanofsky JD. Int J Neurosci 1991, 61, 87-90.

98. Pathogenesis of migraine. Welch KM Semin Neurol 1997, 17, 335-41.

99. Magnesium supplementation as an adjuvant to synthetic calcium channel antagonists in the treatment of hypertension. Touyz RM. Med Hypotheses 1991, 36, 140-1.

100. Ionic basis of hypertension, insulin resistance, vascular disease, and related disorders. The mechanism of "Syndrome X." Resnick LM. Am J Hypertens 1993, 6(4 suppl), 123S-134S.

101. Introduction: Magnesium coming of age. Lauler DP. Sm J Cardiol 1989, 63, 1G-3G.

102. Clinical correlates of the molecular and cellular actions of magnesium on the cardiovascular system. Rienhart RA. Am Heart J 1991, 121(5), 1513-21.

103. Selenium and magnesium status in fibromyalgia. Eisinger J, Plantamura A, Marie PA, Ayavou T. Magnes Res 1994, 7(3-4), 285-8.

104. Increased concentrations of homocysteine in the cerebrospinal fluid inpatients with fibromyalgia and chronic fatigue syndrome. Regland B, Andersson M, Abrahamsson L, Bagby J, Dyrehag LE, Gottfries CG. Scand J Rheumatol 1997, 26(4) 301-307.

105. Viatmin B-12, Vitamin B-6, and folate nutritional status in men with hyperhomocysteinemia. Ubbink JB, Vermaak WJ, van der Merwe A, Becker PJ. Am J Clin Nutr 1993, 57(1), 47-53.

106. Increased concentrations of homocysteine in the cerebrospinal fluid inpatients with fibromyalgia and chronic fatigue syndrome. Regland B, Andersson M, Abrahamsson L, Bagby J, Dyrehag LE, Gottfries CG. Scand J Rheumatol 1997, 26(4) 301-307.

107. Plasma homocysteine in women on oral oestrogen contaning contraceptives and in men with oestrogen treated prostatic carcinoma. Brattstrom L, Israelsson B, Olsson A, Andersson A, Hultberg B. Scand J Clin Lab Invest 1992, 52(4), 283-7.

108. Principles of Biochemistry. Lehninger AL, Nelson DL, Cox MM. Worth Publishers, New York, NY. 1993.

109. Management of fibromyalgia: rationale for the use of magnesium and malic acid. Abraham GE, Flechas JD. J Nutritional Med 1992, 3(1), 49-59.

110. Pain Free. Bucchi LR. The Summit Group. Fort Worth, TX. 1995.

111. Nutrition Applied to Injury Rehabilitation and Sports Medicine. Bucchi LR. CRC Press. Boca Raton, FL. 1995.

112. The discovery of a potent pure chemical wound-healing accelerator. Prudden JF, Migel P, Hanson P, Friedrich L, Balassa L. Am J Surg 1970, 119, 560.

113. Coronary heart disease: reduction of death rate by chondrotin sulfate A. Morrison LM, Enrick NL. Angiology 1973, 24, 269.

114. Effects of hexosamine derivatives and uronic acid derivatives on glycosamineoglycan metabolism of fibroblast cultures. Karzel K, Domenjoz R. Pharmacology 1971, 5, 337.

115. A general practice trial of Ateroid 200 in 8,776 patients with chronic senile cerebral insufficiency. Santini V. Mod Probl Pharmacopsychiatry 1989, 23, 95.

116. Personal communication. Dr. Jacobs is currently preparing a lay publication that will provide detailed descriptions of his observations.

117. The MSM Miracle, Enhance your health with organic sulfur. Earl L. Mindell, R.Ph.,Phd.

118. Indian Medicinal Plants. Kirtikar KR, Basu BD. 1935, 1, 521-9.

119. Boswellin, The Anti-inflammatory Phytonutrient. Majeed M, Badmaev V, Gopinathan S, Rajendran R, Norton T. Nutriscience Publishers, Inc., Piscataway, NJ. 1996.

120. Pharmacology of an extract of salai guggal ex-Boswellia serrata, a new non-steroidal anti-inflammatory agent. Singh GB, Atal CK. Agents Actions 1986, 18, 407-12.

121. Urinary excretion of connective tissue metabolites under the influence of a new non-steroidal anti-inflammatory agent in adjuvant induced arthritis. Kesava Reddy G; Dhar

SC; Singh GB. Agents Actions 1987, 22, 99-105.

122. Application of papaya latex-induced rat paw inflammation: model for evaluation of slowly acting antiarthritic drugs. Gupta OP, Sharma N, Chand D. J Pharmacol Toxicol Methods 1994, 31, 95-8.

123. Urinary excretion of connective tissue metabolites under the influence of a new non-steroidal anti-inflammatory agent in adjuvant induced arthritis. Kesava Reddy G; Dhar SC; Singh GB. Agents Actions 1987, 22, 99-105.

124. Salai Guggal - Boswellia serrata: from a herbal medicine to a non-redox inhibitor of leukotriene biosynthesis. Ammon HP. Eur J Med Res 1996, 1, 369-70.

125. Role of cysteine and glutathione in HIV infection and other diseases associated with muscle wasting and immunological dysfunction. Droege W, Holm E. FASEB Journal 1997, 11(13) 1077-1089.

126. Abnormal glutathione and sulfate levels after interleukin 6 treatment and in tumor-induced cachexia. Hack V, Gross A, Kinscherf R, Bockstette M, Fiers W, Berke G, Droege W. FASEB Journal 1996, 10(10) 1219-1226.

127. Low plasma glutamine in combination with high glutamate levels risk for loss of body cell mass in healthy individuals: The effect of N-acetyl-cysteine. Kinscherf R, Hack V, Fischbach T, Friedmann B, Weiss C, Edler L, Baertsch P, Droege W. J Molecular Med (Berlin) 1996, 74(7), 393-400.

128. N-acetylcysteine inhibits muscle fatigue in humans. Reid MB, Stokic DS, Koch SM, Khawli FA, Leis AA. J Clin Invest 1994, 94(6), 2468-74.

129. Metabolism of cysteine is modified during the acute phase of sepsis in rats. Malmezat T, Breuille D, Pouyet C, Mirand PP, Obled C. J Nutrition 1998, 128(1) 97-105.

130. Role of cysteine and glutathione in HIV infection and other diseases associated with muscle wasting and immunological dysfunction. Droege W, Holm E. FASEB Journal 1997, 11(13) 1077-1089.

131. Evidence for the role of an altered redox state in hyporesponsiveness of synovial T cells in rheumatoid arthritis. Maurice MM; Nakamura H; van der Voort EA; van Vliet AI; Staal FJ; Tak PP; Breedveld FC; Verweij CL. J Immunol 1997, 158, 1458-65.

132. Induction of cytokines and ICAM-1 by proinflammatory cytokines in primary rheumatoid synovial fibroblasts and inhibition by N-acetyl-L-cysteine and aspirin. Sakurada S; Kato T; Okamoto T. Int Immunol 1996, 8, 1483-93.

133. A trial of antioxidants N-acetylcysteine and procysteine in ARDS. The Antioxidant in ARDS Study Group. Bernard GR, Wheeler AP, Arons MM, Morris PE, Paz HL, Russell JA, Wright PE. Chest 1997, 112, 164-72.

134. Circulating antioxidants in ulcerative colitis and their relationship to disease severity and activity. Ramakrishna BS; Varghese R; Jayakumar S; Mathan M; Balasubramanian KA. J Gastroenterol Hepatol 1997, 12, 490-4.

135. Antioxidants and cataract: (cataract induction in space environment and application to terrestrial aging cataract). Bantseev V, Bhardwaj R, Rathbun W, Nagasawa H, Trevithick JR. Biochem Mol Biol Int 1997, 42,1189-97.

136. Suppression of type II collagen-induced arthritis by N-acetyl-L-cysteine in mice. Kroger H, Miesel R, Dietrich A, Ohde M, Altrichter S, Braun C, Ockenfels H. Pharmacol 1997, 29, 671-4.

137. Antioxidants inhibit tumor necrosis factor-alpha mediated stimulation of interleukin-8' monocyte chemoattractant protein-1' and collagenase expression in cultured human synovial cells. Sato M, Miyazaki T, Nagaya T, Murata Y, Ida N, Maeda K, Seo H. J Rheumatol 1996, 23, 432-8.

138. Drug Preparations, Containing Creatine with at Least One Salt of Calcium, Magnesium, Manganese or Zinc. Meyer H. Wo 09800148, Ndn 172-0015-0324-7, 01-08-98.

139. Amine-Secreting Endocrines. Quay WB, Kachi T. In Hormones and Aging, Timiras, PS, Quay WB, Vernadakis A. Eds. CRC Press, Boca Raton. 1995.

140. Melatonin: role in gating nocturnal rise in sleep propensity. Lavie P J Biol Rhythms 1997,

12(6), 657-65.

141. Melatonin and the circadian regulation of sleep initiation' consolidation' structure' and the sleep EEG. Dijk DJ; Cajochen C J Biol Rhythms 1997, 12(6), 627-35.

142. Exogenous melatonin`s phase-shifting effects on the endogenous melatonin profile in sighted humans: a brief review and critique of the literature. Lewy AJ, Sack RL. J Biol Rhythms 1997, 12(6), 588-94.

143. Efficacy of melatonin as a sleep-promoting agent. Zhdanova IV, Wurtman RJ. J Biol Rhythms 1997, 12(6),644-50.

144. Fibromyalgia and migraine, two faces of the same mechanism. Serotonin as the common clue for pathogenesis and therapy. Nicolodi M, Sicuteri F. Adv Exp Med Biol 1996, 398, 73-9.

145. Fibromyalgia and migraine, two faces of the same mechanism. Serotonin as the common clue for pathogenesis and therapy. Nicolodi M, Sicuteri F. Adv Exp Med Biol 1996, 398, 73-9.

146. Primary fibromyalgia syndrome and 5-hydroxy-L-tryptophan: a 90-day open study. Puttini PS, Caruso I. J Int Med Res 1992, 20(2), 182-9.

147. Double-blind study of 5-hydroxytryptophan versus placebo in the treatment of primary fibromyalgia syndrome. Caruso I, Sarzi Puttini P, Cazzola M, Azzolini V. J Int Med Res 1990, 18(3), 201-9.

148. Neuroactive steroids. Paul SM, Purdy RH. FASEB Journal 1992, 6(6), 2311-22.

149. Neurosteroids: of the nervous system, by the nervous system, for the nervous system. Baulieu EE. Recent Prog Horm Res 1997, 520, 1-32.

150. Steroid effects on central neurons and implications for psychiatric and neurological disorders. Holsboer F, Grasser A, Friess E, Wiedemann K. Ann N Y Acad Sci 1994, 7460, 345-59; discussion 359-61.

151. Stress-induced increase in brain neuroactive steroids: antagonism by abercarnil. Barbaccia ML, Roscetti G, Bolacchi F, Concas A, Mostallino MC, Purdy RH, Biggio G. Pharmacol Biochem Behav 1996, 54(1),:205-10.

152. Evidence for adrenocortical adaptation to severe illness. Parker LN, Levin ER, Lifrak ET. J Clin Endocrinol Metab 1985, 60(5), 947-52.

153. [Adrenal cortical function in chronic diseases.] Goncharova ND, Goncharov NP. Source Probl Endokrinol (Mosk) 1988, 34(6), 27-31.

154. Acute and chronic methyl mercury poisoning impairs rat adrenal and testicular function. Burton GV, Meikle AW. J Toxicol Environ Health 1980, 6(3), 597-606.

155. Differential anxiolytic effects of neurosteroids in the mirrored chamber behavior test in mice. Reddy DS, Kulkarni SK. Brain Res 1997, 752(1-2), 61-71.

156. Neurosteroid pregnenolone induces sleep-EEG changes in man compatible with inverse agonist GABAA-receptor modulation. Steiger A, Trachsel L, Guldner J, Hemmeter U, Rothe, B, Rupprecht R, Vedder H, Holsboer F. Brain Res 1993, 615, 267-274.

157. Biologically active and other chemical constituents of the herb of Hypericum perforatum L. Nahrstedt A, Butterweck V. Pharmacopsychiatry 1997, 30(Suppl 20),129-34.

158. Controlled clinical trials of hypericum extracts in depressed patients—an overview. Volz HP. Pharmacopsychiatry 1997, 30(Suppl 20), 72-6.

159. Efficacy and tolerability of St. John`s wort extract LI 160 versus imipramine in patients with severe depressive episodes according to ICD-10. Vorbach EU, Arnoldt KH, Hubner WD. Pharmacopsychiatry 1997, 30(Suppl 20), 81-5.

160. LI 160' an extract of St. John`s wort' versus amitriptyline in mildly to moderately depressed outpatients—a controlled 6-week clinical trial. Wheatley D. Pharmacopsychiatry 1997, 30(Suppl 20), 77-80.

161. Treatment of seasonal affective disorder (SAD) with hypericum extract. Kasper S. Pharmacopsychiatry 1997, 30(Suppl 20), 89-93.

162. [Pharmacotherapy.] Laux G. Ther Umsch 1997, 54(10), 595-9.

163. [Effect of a special kava extract in patients with anxiety, tension, and excitation states of non-psychotic genesis. Double blind study with placebos over 4 weeks.] Kinzler E, Kromer J, Lehmann E. Arzneimittelforschung 1991, 41(6), 584-8.

164. Kava-kava extract WS 1490 versus placebo in anxiety disorders—a randomized placebo-controlled 25-week outpatient trial. Volz HP, Kieser M. Pharmacopsychiatry 1997, 30(1), 1-5.

165. [Psychosomatic dysfunctions in the female climacteric. Clinical effectiveness and tolerance of Kava Extract WS 1490.] Warnecke G. Fortschr Med 1991, 109(4), 119-22.

166. Kava: an overview. Singh YN. J Ethnopharmacol 1992, 37(1), 13-45.

167. The prevalence of chronic widespread pain in the general population. Croft P, Rigby AS, Boswell R, Schollum J, Silman A. J Rheumatol 1993, 20, 710-3.

168. Fibromyalgia and the rheumatisms. Common sense and sensibility. Block SR. Rheum Dis Clin North Am 1993, 19(1), 61-78.